## Co-occurring Disorders Series

# UNDERSTANDING MAJOR ANXIETY DISORDERS AND ADDICTION

Revised

### Katie Evans, Ph.D.

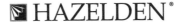 HAZELDEN®

FORMERLY THE DUAL DIAGNOSIS SERIES

Hazelden
Center City, Minnesota 55012-0176

1-800-328-9000
1-651-213-4590 (Fax)
www.hazelden.org

To request permission, write to
Permissions Coordinator, Hazelden
P.O. Box 176, Center City, MN 55012-0176.
To purchase additional copies of this publication, call
1-800-328-9000 or 1-651-213-4000.

ISBN: 1-59285-017-0

**Editor's note**

This material was written to educate individuals about chemical dependency
and mental illness. It is not intended as a substitute for professional medical
or psychiatric care.

Any stories or case studies that may be used in this material are com-
posites of many individuals. Names and details have been changed to protect
identities.

The Twelve Steps are reprinted and adapted with permission of Alcoholics
Anonymous World Services, Inc. Permission to reprint and adapt the Twelve
Steps does not mean that Alcoholics Anonymous (AA) has reviewed or
approved the contents of this publication, nor that AA agrees with the views
expressed herein. The views expressed herein are solely those of the author. AA
is a program of recovery from alcoholism. Use of the Twelve Steps in connec-
tion with programs and activities that are patterned after AA, but that address
other problems, does not imply otherwise.

Cover and interior design by Lightbourne

# CONTENTS

*To my children, Casey and Callie, for their love and support. For all the dual disorder individuals who have taught me most of what I know.*

# INTRODUCTION

This is written for you, the person suffering from two diseases: chemical dependency and a major anxiety disorder. You may be surprised to learn that a major anxiety disorder is a disease just like cancer, Alzheimer's, chemical dependency, diabetes, or many other medical problems. Maybe you're reading this because you or someone close to you is concerned about your high levels of anxiety. Perhaps a psychiatrist, physician, psychologist, or other qualified professional has said that you suffer from a major anxiety disorder. Or you could be one of the thousands of recovering alcoholics or addicts who are working a Twelve Step program of recovery, yet continue to suffer from a high level of fear, tension, and worry and still have a hard time living life on life's terms. This may have led you to consider taking that first drink or pill. You may have even considered giving up, thinking that the program is just not working for you.

This pamphlet was written to help you work a combined recovery program for both your chemical dependency and your anxiety disorder. Information will be given to you about your dual disorder and some practical suggestions will be offered for working a combined program. This material will help you to develop and maintain pro-recovery attitudes and to take action to get out of the problem and into the solution. This pamphlet is *not* a quick fix or a substitute for professional

Duplicating this page is illegal. Do not copy this material without written permission from the publisher.

1

assistance. It *is* a source of ideas and tools with which to complement other parts of your recovery program.

The term "dual disorders" refers to two or more co-occurring disorders. This pamphlet will discuss chemical addiction and major anxiety disorders. The question of which came first—the anxiety or the addiction—is irrelevant since both disorders can jeopardize your recovery and emotional sobriety.

This pamphlet will emphasize the importance of working a comprehensive dual recovery program.

People who are severely anxious can become chemically dependent and people who are chemically dependent people can suffer from severe anxiety. Anxiety is common when someone is either actively using alcohol or other drugs or is in early recovery from addiction. Using mood-altering chemicals for long periods can actually increase your feelings of anxiety. Part of the increase is due to your body's response to the chemicals themselves; part is your attempt to "manage the unmanageable." Perhaps you are trying to remain in control not only of your chemical use, but also of people, places, and things.

Even as you enter recovery and abstain from alcohol and other drugs, you may experience some serious anxiety. Some of these feelings are withdrawal symptoms. The realization of what your drinking and using has done to your life can be overwhelming. What addict wouldn't feel anxious and overwhelmed to learn that he or she could no longer drink and use? It makes sense that you feel anxious and overwhelmed if you've come to depend on chemicals for answers to your problems. You are not as in control as you thought, and you now must face the task of cleaning up the damage of your past. You can expect to feel anxious at times during the first few weeks and months of abstinence. But the anxiety should gradually diminish after you are free of chemicals, as you maintain abstinence, and as you start working a Twelve Step program.

This pamphlet focuses on the anxiety disorders that, if left untreated, last beyond the weeks and months of staying clean and sober and working a recovery program. These include panic, obsessive-compulsive, and generalized anxiety disorders. (Post-traumatic stress disorder, which is also considered a major anxiety disorder, is somewhat different from the disorders discussed here. It has been treated separately in this pamphlet series.) These disorders can dilute the quality of your recovery from chemical dependency, lead to a relapse into drinking or using other drugs, or even make suicide seem attractive.

By learning how to work a program for both your chemical dependency and your anxiety disorder, you will begin to experience the serenity that others working a Twelve Step program have found. And you will experience the Promises offered in the Big Book of Alcoholics Anonymous (AA).[*]

> Appendix A, page 33, contains questions that you can answer to increase your understanding of the material in this pamphlet. Appendix B, page 35, provides a chart to help you develop a daily schedule of activities. Appendix C, page 37, is a list of useful Twelve Step slogans.

---

[*] The Promises of the rewards that come with working a recovery program appear throughout *Alcoholics Anonymous* (published by Alcoholics Anonymous World Services, Inc., New York, 3d ed., 1976); see especially the last paragraph on page 83 through line 15 on page 84.

# THE DISEASES OF CHEMICAL DEPENDENCY AND MAJOR ANXIETY DISORDERS

Chemical dependency and anxiety disorders are two separate diseases. Table 1, below, outlines the causes, symptoms, and necessary steps in working a successful recovery program. Table 2, page 7, outlines the progression and the recovery process typical of both chemical dependency and anxiety disorders. These tables and the following discussion will help you understand your dual disorders and your recovery program.

Table 1

| COMPARISON OF THE DISEASES OF CHEMICAL DEPENDENCY AND MAJOR ANXIETY DISORDERS (Panic, Obsessive-Compulsive, and Generalized Anxiety Disorders) | | |
|---|---|---|
| **Factor** | **Chemical Dependency** | **Major Anxiety Disorder** |
| *Causes* | • alcohol and other drug use | • stress and threatened loss of significant relationships, achievements, and status |

Table 1 *(continued)*

| Factor | Chemical Dependency | Major Anxiety Disorder |
|---|---|---|
| *Causes (continued)* | • changes in brain chemistry and brain function<br><br>• hereditary and environmental factors | • changes in brain chemistry and brain function<br><br>• hereditary and environmental factors |
| *Symptoms* | • tolerance, withdrawal, progression<br><br>• denial<br>• loss of control<br><br>• continued use despite negative consequences<br>• physical, interpersonal, social, occupational, spiritual problems<br>• hospitalization, imprisonment, insanity, death | • muscle tension and overactive bodily responses: pounding heart, trembling, etc.<br>• hypervigilance<br>• severe anxiety and worry<br>• avoidance of feared situations<br>• physical, interpersonal, social, occupational, spiritual problems<br>• hospitalization, immobilization, suicide |
| *Recovery Program* | • abstinence<br>• Twelve Step meeting attendance<br><br>• sponsor<br>• Step work through reading recovery materials and helping others | • social support<br>• relaxation skills and gradual approach to feared situations<br><br>• constructive thinking<br>• medication and/or psychotherapy |

Table 2

# HOW MAJOR ANXIETY DISORDERS AND ADDICTION PROGRESS AND HOW YOU CAN RECOVER

**Downward Progression**

nervousness
increased tension
worry and overanalyzing
increased physical symptoms
agitation
anxiety attacks
avoidance of feared situations
excessive vigilance
rituals
confusion
family problems
work or school problems
severe anxiety
depression
thoughts of suicide

**Recovery**

achieves serenity
employer confidence grows
family relations improve
functions better overall
faces dreaded situations
eats right
gets physical exercise
starts positive thinking
learns relaxation skills
may need medication
turns worry over to Higher Power
seeks support from others
begins to work program
accepts diseases
learn assertiveness
and boundary setting

**Recovery Program**

# The Disease of Chemical Dependency

If you drink alcohol or take other drugs that have abuse potential, you can start a process of change in your brain chemistry. Eventually the result can be addiction. If you have a family history of alcoholism or other addictions, the chances are greater that this process will occur in you. *Tolerance* means that you need to take increasing amounts of a substance to achieve the same effects. It is one sign that the physical process of addiction has begun. Another sign is *withdrawal,* which means that after you stop drinking or using, you will feel very uncomfortable. Physical, mental, and emotional problems can develop. Withdrawal can be life threatening, especially with alcohol, tranquilizers, and other sedatives, and requires medical management.

Other key symptoms of the disease of chemical dependency are *loss of control* and *continued use of chemicals* despite the serious problems they cause. Perhaps you have tried to cut down on your use—or even quit—but you cannot. Maybe you find that you keep drinking or using more than you had planned. Another symptom, *progression,* means taking more and more of the substance for longer periods of time and/or using more of different kinds of addictive substances. Maybe you find you have become so preoccupied with chemical use that using has become the most important thing in your life—more important than other activities and people. Perhaps you continue to use despite damage to your body, fights at home, problems on the job, legal problems, or loss of faith and hope. These are all symptoms of the disease of chemical dependency.

*Denial* is strong in the disease of chemical dependency. No doubt you felt denial before you entered recovery. You have a disease that says you don't have a disease! Blaming others is part of denial, and so is making excuses for your drinking and using and the problems they have caused.

Chemical dependency is a *progressive disease*—that is, it gets worse with time, if not treated. It is a chronic disease that has no cure. But you can experience a remission, a reduction of your symptoms. Recovery starts with abstinence from all mood-altering chemicals. You can get the support and guidance you need to promote your recovery by attending Alcoholics Anonymous or similar Twelve Step self-help groups and by working with a Twelve Step sponsor to guide you into recovery. Working the Steps can lead you to accept your disease. It can help you repair the emotional and spiritual damage caused by your drinking and using. You will learn that you are sick getting well, not bad getting good.

## Major Anxiety Disorders

It is important to understand that a major anxiety disorder is a disease just as chemical dependency is a disease. This means that if you suffer from an anxiety disorder, you are sick getting well, not bad getting good. You are not responsible for the disorder. But you are responsible for working a good recovery program for your disorder.

Sometimes an anxiety disorder seems to come out of nowhere. And sometimes it's something you've experienced for so long that you aren't sure when you didn't have it. Sometimes a major loss or the threat of one can trigger an anxiety disorder; for example, the death of a parent or spouse, a divorce, or losing a job. Ongoing stress, such as fights with your spouse, work problems, or tough financial circumstances, can trigger an anxiety disorder too. Also, if you have family members with an anxiety disorder, you are at high risk for developing one yourself.

When you experience anxiety, do you notice that you

are shaky or tense? Do you get restless or tired easily? Perhaps you are short of breath or feel as if you're being smothered. Do you have hot, sweaty hands or cold, clammy ones? Are you dizzy and light-headed at times, or do you get nausea and diarrhea? Perhaps you have hot flashes or chills, or a dry mouth and trouble swallowing. All of these are physical signs of your disorder.

There are other signs too. You may have trouble concentrating or you may feel your mind go blank. You may feel on edge and startle easily. You may have trouble sleeping or feel constantly irritable. You may have thoughts you don't want and can't stop thinking. You may experience fear that you might go crazy, lose control, or die.

You may find yourself avoiding situations that you fear will provoke anxiety. Or you may take extreme measures to keep anxiety at bay—even if it means you no longer carry out your daily activities. Perhaps you avoid crossing certain bridges or stay at home all the time and away from public places, or perhaps you go out only with a companion. Perhaps you have repeated thoughts of violence toward loved ones, fear harmless situations, or can't be sure whether you've performed some act. Maybe you perform certain rituals, such as constantly washing your hands, counting, checking the stove, or touching your face. Perhaps you can no longer do household chores or go to work. Possibly you no longer enjoy time with family and friends, and fights with them may have gotten worse. You may even have become so depressed that you think about suicide.

Thinking too hard and overanalyzing are part of early recovery and an anxiety disorder. You may scan your surroundings or monitor your body, ever alert to signs of danger. You may also be at the ready to escape from situations that trigger intense discomfort. Your anxiety can even increase if the signs you feared turn out to be false alarms. Perhaps you have become preoccupied with "just-in-case" thinking, doing and thinking of all kinds of distressing things just in case danger lies ahead. You are living in tomorrow instead of one day at a time.

If you suffer from a *panic disorder,* you experience unexpected and unpredictable periods of intense fear or discomfort. Sometimes they last minutes and sometimes hours. You may have developed agoraphobia, a strong fear of being in situations that make escape difficult or embarrassing or where help might not be available. Sometimes the panic attacks are limited and agoraphobia is the predominant problem. If you suffer from an *obsessive-compulsive* disorder, you may try to avoid unwanted and senseless thoughts or impulses. This disorder may lead you to repeat actions (rituals) that are designed to prevent some dreaded event or situation. If you have a *generalized anxiety disorder,* you may suffer intense and constant anxiety and worry about all sorts of things; this kind of anxiety doesn't simply occur from time to time but is of long duration.

## The Role of Codependency

There are many definitions of codependency. The preferred one here is this: Someone making other people's needs so important that their own needs don't get met.

Codependency can certainly cause anxiety. If you suffer from codependency, you often put your self-esteem in the hands of others—you have more respect for others' opinions than for your own. Constantly asking questions such as "Do you think I should quit my job?" is one example.

Codependency can accompany an anxiety disorder. For instance, you have an anxiety disorder that causes you to worry a lot. Your spouse may become a focus of your worry. In trying to get rid of your worry, you may try to change his or her behavior. Trying to control another person's behavior can be extremely frustrating and nerve-wracking—which causes you more anxiety. This attempt at control is a symptom of codependency.

Codependency can also look like an anxiety disorder. Perhaps you are living with a practicing alcoholic. Over time you have become as focused on the drinking as your spouse has. Worrying about "what if" he kills someone while driving drunk or "what if" she gets arrested can lead you to intervene by hiding his car keys or "misplacing" her wallet. All of this worry and stress leads to intense feelings of anxiety. The key to recovery from codependency lies in learning to let go of trying to control the behavior of other people. Be kind to yourself.

## Kathy's Story

Kathy, who was working a Twelve Step recovery program, had been sober for six months when she experienced her first panic attack. She had been taking on a lot, trying to make up for lost time during her drinking and using days.

Being she was the mother of two small children, Kathy tried to help out with the household finances by doing day care in her home. In addition to baby-sitting, Kathy had volunteered to raise money for the March of Dimes and was organizing a clothing drive for her church. She felt overwhelmed at times but scolded herself, thinking, *It's not like I am working full time!* Kathy was a perfectionist, so she felt she had to do all her tasks the best and most complete way.

About four o'clock one afternoon, Kathy began to feel more anxious than usual. Her heart started pounding, her pulse began racing, and she became frozen with unexplained fear. She was breathing abnormally fast and couldn't move for about twenty minutes. She nearly passed out. Kathy had experienced her first panic attack.

She tried to discuss her "stressed out" episode with her husband. Bill, who was preoccupied with his own business problems, told Kathy that she just needed to learn to "chill out and relax" and not to take things so seriously. This feedback led Kathy to feel she was somehow a weak person who couldn't handle life like other people she had met in her AA meetings. Kathy's guilt and shame increased, so did the frequency of her panic attacks.

She began discussing her panic attacks with a supportive friend who was also in recovery. Her friend suggested she practice the Twelve Steps on both her anxiety and addiction. Finally, feeling desperate one day, Kathy called a therapist recommended to her by her AA friend. Kathy learned that she had a major anxiety disorder—a disease—in addition to her chemical dependency. Her therapist referred her to a physician knowledgeable about the problems of people who are chemically dependent. He prescribed BuSpar, a nonaddictive antianxiety medication, and the panic attacks soon subsided.

With her therapist, Kathy began to learn relaxation techniques as well as to deal with her strong need for approval from her husband. She came to understand her codependency and the fear of abandonment she had felt since childhood as the result of growing up in an alcoholic family. Kathy learned to accept that she wasn't "weak" or "bad" but was, in fact, in recovery from two diseases.

## Recovery Is Attainable

Recovery from either the disease of chemical addiction or an anxiety disorder is often challenging. And recovery from an addiction is especially hard if you suffer from periods of overwhelming anxiety. But recovery *is* possible, and understanding and accepting that you are suffering from coexisting disorders is the beginning of your journey of recovery.

The next section will discuss the steps you can take to begin your combined recovery program.

# HOW TO WORK A COMBINED PROGRAM OF RECOVERY

In this section, effective strategies for working a combined program of recovery from your dual disorders of chemical dependency and a major anxiety disorder will be discussed. Table 2, page 7, shows both progression of, and recovery from, these disorders.

## A Recovery Program

Recovery from chemical dependency requires that you accept your disease of chemical dependency and abstain from mood-altering chemicals. It also involves attending Twelve Step meetings, getting a sponsor, working the Twelve Steps, and improving your physical health.

Recovery from a major anxiety disorder also requires that you accept your disease. It involves seeking support from others and learning to relax and think constructively. It requires a shift in thinking from being fear based to faith based.

## Acceptance

It is crucial that you accept the dual diseases of chemical

dependency and an anxiety disorder. Without *acceptance,* you are likely to deny having any problem or to remain trapped in the idea that you are weak or bad. You might still think that you could get better if only you tried hard enough. If you review the symptoms outlined in the last section and see how they apply to you, you will begin to understand that you are not weak but that you have two diseases. Acceptance of your disorders is the first step in recovery.

## Abstinence

You must be abstinent from addictive, mood-altering chemicals. Using alcohol, tranquilizers, sedatives, or other mood-altering chemicals will make both of your diseases worse and will prevent the process of recovery from beginning. Without *abstinence,* you will be unable to control your use of chemicals. You will continue to experience life problems as a result of your addiction that affect your body, mind, and behavior. Your anxiety will continue to remain high and even increase; your efforts to deal with it will fail. As you continue to feel out of control and avoid facing your fears directly, your denial and worry will increase. Abstinence, however, can help you develop new solutions to your old problems.

Keep in mind that there are nonaddictive medications such as antidepressants that may be recommended to help restore important brain chemistry.

## An Active Recovery Program

Just as your dual diseases have dominated your life and made it unmanageable, you now need to make a priority of working an *active recovery program.* Merely abstaining from chemicals and waiting around for your anxiety to disappear will guarantee continued unhappiness and problems in living. In a word, recovery depends not on what you *won't* do, but on what you *will* do. Positive thinking will help to turn things over and will lead to faith.

## Support from Others

*Attending Twelve Step meetings,* such as Alcoholics Anonymous (AA), Narcotics Anonymous (NA), or Cocaine Anonymous (CA), will serve as a key support as you stay clean and sober and address your anxiety. At these meetings, you will hear others share their experiences, strengths, and hopes. You will find fellowship with those who have struggled and still struggle with many of the same issues you face. You can talk honestly about your problems and feelings and efforts to recover without fear of judgment, ridicule, or criticism. The open, caring, and nonjudgmental atmosphere of Twelve Step meetings will help you combat your feelings of being bad and shameful. These meetings will help you practice expressing your thoughts and feelings directly in a safe place. Members may offer supportive comments after the meeting and offer to talk with you on the phone. Most areas have different groups meeting at different times, so you will always have a place to go for support.

Besides this general support, *obtaining a sponsor* is helpful. Sponsors are members of a Twelve Step group who act as mentors and guides. They help you learn about Twelve Step programs and support you during those tough times when you feel alone and believe that nobody understands how you feel.

Of course, getting out to meetings can be hard when you're feeling anxious and overwhelmed. This is especially true if you experience social anxiety or agoraphobia, which involves fear of being with strangers. It also can involve fear of being in situations where you might be embarrassed if you showed symptoms of anxiety or where you would find escape difficult. But you do have some options. Perhaps a family member or friend could accompany you to meetings. Or you could call the local AA or NA office and ask that someone come to your home to make a Twelfth Step visit. As you work the other parts of your recovery program, you will feel more comfortable about going out. Taking small steps one day at a time keeps you on your path to recovery.

## Taking Care of Yourself

If you *practice relaxation techniques,* you can diminish the physical symptoms of your anxiety and thus strengthen your recovery program. Most bookstores sell books that give detailed instructions for learning these skills. Usually this involves learning to breathe properly and to relax your muscles. Practice breathing in slowly and deeply from your stomach and through your nose, then slowly exhaling and relaxing all your muscles; do this several times in a row. Practice this several times a day when you are least anxious. Gradually, you'll be able to relax your body on command.

Go bowling, take a brisk walk, or ride a bicycle (even a stationary one at home). Yoga, meditation, and prayer can also prove very helpful in working a dual recovery program. These *physical activities* will help you to relax and will promote a sense of well-being. They provide alternatives to drinking and using. Exercise also helps repair the distorted brain chemistry that can result from your dual disorders.

*Developing a weekly schedule* is a good idea. With a schedule, you'll have external structure to help you keep a good balance of work, play, and social activities as well as to ensure an active recovery program. Allow for rest and self-care. Fill out a schedule for Sunday through Saturday, from 8 A.M. to midnight, blocking out times for your activities. Be sure to fill any holes in your schedule that are left open. Appendix B, page 35, contains a sample blank schedule.

*Maintaining good nutrition* is helpful. Developing and sticking to a food plan that includes proper amounts of the basic food groups is a good start. Foods with complex carbohydrates (fruits, vegetables, cereals, and grains) are especially good for promoting a more relaxed feeling. Eating right will help supply essential nutrients that have been reduced in value by stress and your use of chemicals. You need these nutrients for physical energy, clear thinking, and the emotional staying power necessary to deal with life's challenges. Lots of books and articles on good nutrition are available in libraries and bookstores.

## Thinking Constructively

Alcohol and other drug abuse often distorts your thinking. It can cause denial and other attitudes that lead you to make excuses for your problems. Your anxiety disorder can also distort your thinking. It can lead to a view of the world that says you are in danger and at the mercy of mysterious and powerful forces. You then become excessively alert, fearful of even the slightest hint of a dreaded situation. You may become so afraid of experiencing any anxiety at all that even innocent situations can cause alarms to go off. In combination with being constantly alert, you may be constantly ready to take any action to avoid dreaded situations, no matter how distressing they are to you and to others. "Watch out," "On stage," "Be prepared," and "Disaster plan in effect" are likely to be constant refrains in your thinking. A particular danger for a person who is chemically dependent is the belief that "only one drink or pill will help me relax, so I'll take one just in case." Feeling that you are the exception to the rule is another problem.

The theme of all this thinking is managing the unmanageable. By attempting to control both your chemical use and the sources of your anxiety, you end up not only failing to fix the problem, but also making things worse. The more you think you can control it all, the worse it all becomes.

Members of Twelve Step groups use certain phrases, called slogans, to express helpful ways to view themselves and the world. Some examples are "Sick getting well, not bad getting good," "One day at a time," and "Let go and let God." You'll find more Twelve Step slogans in appendix C, page 37. *Saying these slogans* to yourself when you feel wound up, in danger, and overwhelmed will help you cultivate acceptance and serenity. You can also include a review of the slogans in your daily schedule once or twice a day and focus on one that seems particularly meaningful to you at that moment. At first this may seem artificial, but with repetition and practice you are likely to experience a slow but sure change in your anxious thinking.

## Working the Twelve Steps

Part of a combined recovery program is *working the Twelve Steps* as a program for living. Not only can Twelve Step work help you maintain a chemically free lifestyle, it can also aid you in achieving peace of mind by helping you cope with the stresses and problems in your life. On the next page is the complete Twelve Steps of Alcoholics Anonymous.

## The Twelve Steps of Alcoholics Anonymous*

1. We admitted we were powerless over alcohol—that our lives had become unmanageable.

2. Came to believe that a Power greater than ourselves could restore us to sanity.

3. Made a decision to turn our will and our lives over to the care of God *as we understood Him.*

4. Made a searching and fearless moral inventory of ourselves.

5. Admitted to God, to ourselves, and to another human being the exact nature of our wrongs.

6. Were entirely ready to have God remove all these defects of character.

7. Humbly asked Him to remove our shortcomings.

8. Made a list of all persons we had harmed, and became willing to make amends to them all.

9. Made direct amends to such people wherever possible, except when to do so would injure them or others.

10. Continued to take personal inventory and when we were wrong promptly admitted it.

11. Sought through prayer and meditation to improve our conscious contact with God *as we understood Him,* praying only for knowledge of His will for us and the power to carry that out.

12. Having had a spiritual awakening as the result of these steps, we tried to carry this message to alcoholics, and to practice these principles in all our affairs.

---

* The Twelve Steps of Alcoholics Anonymous are taken from *Alcoholics Anonymous,* 3d ed., published by Alcoholics Anonymous World Services, Inc., New York, NY., pages 59–60. Reprinted with permission of Alcoholics Anonymous World Services, Inc. The synopsis that immediately follows the listing of the Twelve Steps is not a part of the Twelve Steps; it consists of comments by the author of this pamphlet.

Step One is the foundation of your recovery program from chemical dependency: acknowledging your powerlessness over alcohol and/or drugs and the problems that they have caused. For recovery from your anxiety disorder, the foundation is admitting that you are powerless over your obsessive thoughts and attempts to control other people, places, and things.

Step Two is a faith Step. It gives you hope that things are improving and that there is a Power greater than yourself that can help you recover.

Step Three teaches you to let go of obsessive thinking and your attempts to control everything. Turning your worry over to a Higher Power can be a great source of both support and peace of mind.

Steps Four and Five offer you a chance to get a more realistic picture of yourself. Some of us have low self-esteem and think, *No one is as bad as I am!* Some of us are a little self-centered and have an exaggerated idea of our own importance. Steps Four and Five give you a chance to see realistically who you are. This includes your attributes and shortcomings.

Steps Six through Twelve help you become less centered on yourself and more concerned with being helpful to others. They help you live in the solution instead of in the problem.

## Facing Fears

A difficult but crucial part of recovery from your anxiety disorder is facing your fears directly. Right now, you may be holding on to your anxiety by escaping dreaded situations—either by avoiding them or by using chemicals, rituals, or other means. *Gradually working through your anxiety and fear* is important. You must no longer avoid anxiety-provoking situations. What you must now avoid is escape.

You may be thinking, *But I can't!* Remember that you now have others available to support you, that you have learned new ways to relax, and that you can work on a new set of attitudes to help you cope. Remember, too, that you can do this step by step. Perhaps you will start by walking alone in the yard. Maybe you'll decide to worry about things only three times a day for a total of a half hour. Or maybe you'll try to say hello to that familiar person at the meeting. Although this may be intensely uncomfortable at the outset, you will fast discover two things: first, that you can tolerate the anxiety, and second, that your anxiety will gradually disappear. As contradictory as it may seem, by allowing yourself to be anxious, you will ultimately gain serenity. In Twelve Step programs, FEAR is defined as "False Evidence Appearing Real."

## Getting Psychotherapy

*Psychotherapy* with a qualified professional can be a very useful part of your combined recovery program. A psychotherapist can give you support. He or she can help you organize and stick to a recovery plan, teach you new ways to handle self-defeating thoughts and actions, and help you work through intense feelings.

If you aren't in the care of one already, it's recommended that you look for a licensed or certified mental health professional. Look for one experienced in both mental health and chemical dependency. Talk with people in your Twelve Step meetings or call recovery centers to get a referral. In your first session with a therapist, be sure to ask whether he or she has expertise in addiction recovery as well as anxiety disorders.

While psychotherapy alone is no substitute for the other things you need to do, it can complement your recovery work.

# THREE

# MEDICATION

A major anxiety disorder is a disease, and certain kinds of medication can be very helpful in your recovery. Medication can help the bodily symptoms of anxiety, such as muscle tension and hot flashes. It can even help with bothersome, unwanted worry. It's hard to work your program if you're constantly keyed up. Taking medication can complement the other parts of the recovery program talked about in the previous section. It can be especially useful if you experience constant, high levels of anxiety or if other strategies don't seem to work for you. But medications can mean special problems for people who are also chemically dependent. This must be clearly and closely evaluated.

## Sam's Story

Sam had anxiety attacks as far back as he could remember. When he went to college, his anxiety got so high that he would freeze with fear, making it hard for him to participate in class or social activities or to take exams. He got help from his family doctor in the form of tranquilizers, with the instructions to use them only when he got very nervous. But it didn't take long before he began to rely heavily on the pills, just in case he should begin to feel anxious.

But then Sam noticed his pills weren't lasting very

long. Since he was embarrassed to tell his doctor how many he was taking, he got a second prescription from the college infirmary. He began to take two pills instead of one because one just didn't seem to work anymore.

One night at a college fraternity party, Sam drank whiskey after having taken some pills. He fell unconscious and was rushed to a hospital emergency room. The doctors stabilized his condition, then transferred him to the hospital's alcohol and drug treatment unit. There Sam began therapy for his addiction to tranquilizers.

In the early days of his recovery, Sam was extremely anxious. He feared that his anxiety attacks would return with their old regularity. A physician from the alcohol and drug treatment unit, understanding the problems of dual disorders, prescribed a nonaddictive antidepressant medication for his anxiety. And Sam's counselor in the unit suggested he begin to work the Twelve Steps for both his chemical dependency and his anxiety disorder. Before long, Sam was successfully working a combined program of recovery from his two diseases.

## Special Concerns for the Person

## Who Is Chemically Dependent

Recovering from chemical dependency presents a problem if you are considering the use of medication for an anxiety disorder. If recovery requires abstinence from mood-altering chemicals, how can you justify taking medications used for anxiety disorders that are themselves mood-altering?

Remember that you have coexisting disorders, addiction and a major anxiety disorder. Try to distinguish between a chemical you abuse and a medication you take to treat a disease. Recall, too, that Alcoholics Anonymous and similar recovery groups have no official position on medication. Rather, they urge their members to consult physicians on such issues. It is always important to be honest in discussing with your physician both your addiction and your concerns regarding the abuse potential of *any* medication. It is especially helpful to have a doctor who is familiar and comfortable with Twelve Step recovery.

## Types of Medications

Medical professionals use a variety of medications to treat an anxiety disorder. Some are safe for the person recovering from chemical dependency and some are risky. Antidepressant medications, for example, are often effective for anxiety disorders; they have little abuse potential and are not addictive.

But be aware that some medications prescribed for anxiety disorders *can* be addictive. These are the benzo-diazepine-based medications such as Valium and Xanax. They have effects similar to those of alcohol and are in fact a category of "depressant" drugs. These tranquilizers, as well as another class of drugs known as sedative-hypnotics, can be abused and can cause serious addiction. BuSpar is an antianxiety medication that, so far, has not been addictive in a variety of tests. On the other hand, the early reports that some tranquilizers weren't addictive proved wrong. Time will tell about BuSpar.

Tell your doctor that you do *not* wish to take any medication with potential for addiction. At the same time, rest assured that antidepressant medications are generally safe for the person in recovery.

## Taking Your Medication

Antidepressant medications do have some limitations.

They take several weeks to become effective. They can have side effects such as drowsiness, a decrease in blood pressure, dizziness, dry mouth, blurred vision, and constipation. And they don't work for everyone.

But don't let their limitations scare you off. Support from your family, friends, doctor, and Twelve Step sponsor can help you get through the several weeks that may be needed before the medication becomes effective. Many side effects disappear as your body gets used to the medication. Your doctor can also determine the best dose for you, one that is effective yet minimizes side effects.

Remember to take your medication only as prescribed. *Always* consult your physician about a change in dose and *never* stop taking your medication without talking to your doctor. Suddenly stopping some antidepressant medications can cause reactions such as nausea, nightmares, or agitation. Don't get caught in the trap of thinking, *I feel fine now, so obviously I don't need the medication anymore.* Your medication is very likely part of what's helping you feel better. Maintain your motivation by seeking support from others. And combine medication with the other strategies in the previous section.

## Emily's Story

Emily found that as hard as she tried, she just couldn't seem to work her program of recovery from chemical dependency. Worry and agitation kept her awake at night. She felt tired and irritated all day and nervous in the evenings. While at AA meetings Emily felt good, but by the time she got home, she had begun to get anxious again. Often she felt nauseated or had diarrhea.

Emily discussed her situation with her AA sponsor, who suggested that she see a psychiatrist who was an expert at treating addictions. So Emily took her sponsor's advice and went to see Dr. Spencer. Aware that Emily was recovering from chemical dependency, Dr. Spencer prescribed an antidepressant medication that Emily could take at bedtime. After a couple of weeks, Emily began to sleep through the night. This helped improve her mood.

Emily also began to think about HALTS, the word Alcoholics Anonymous uses as a reminder of triggers for relapse. She remembered that the initials stand for **H**ungry, **A**ngry, **L**onely, **T**ired, and **S**ick. Emily could see that her anxiety had probably been the cause of the nausea and diarrhea, and she certainly had been very tired due to lack of sleep. With Dr. Spencer's help, she began to learn how to take better care of herself physically and emotionally. After a month of working with Dr. Spencer and using antidepressants, Emily was able to turn her worries over to a Higher Power when she began to worry too much. The medication had an important role in helping her work a combined program of recovery.

# IN CLOSING

I hope you now begin to know and accept that you suffer from two diseases: chemical dependency and a major anxiety disorder.

While we are not responsible for *having* our diseases and the problems they bring to our lives, we are responsible for *finding solutions* to recovering from them.

Working a combined program of recovery for your dual disorders can help guide you out of the problem and into the solution, one day at a time.

# APPENDIX A

# COMING TO KNOW
# YOUR DISORDERS

Use this worksheet to help apply the information in this pamphlet to your life. After you read the pamphlet, take some time to write down your answers for each item below. You may also wish to review your answers with your sponsor, your therapist, a friend, or an appropriate family member.

1. Write down at least five signs or problems that indicate that you suffer from the disease of chemical dependency.

2. Write down at least five signs or problems that indicate that you suffer from the disease of a major anxiety disorder.

3. Explain why you are "sick getting well," not "bad getting good," and why you are not responsible for having the diseases of chemical dependency and major anxiety.

4. List any major reservations you may have about accepting your two diseases. For each reservation, list one thing you could think or do to deal with this reservation.

5. List any major roadblocks that might stop you from making active recovery a priority in your life. Consider such obstacles as money and time, an

unsupportive spouse, and your own attitudes. (For example, you don't believe recovery will make a difference.) For each roadblock, list a possible solution.

6. Explain why abstinence from alcohol and drugs is necessary for your recovery from both disorders.

7. List at least three things you could do to promote your recovery from your chemical dependency. Do the same for your major anxiety disorder.

8. Describe any concerns you may have about taking medication for your anxiety disorder. Then for each, describe how you might resolve this concern.

9. Describe several ways that counseling or therapy could help your recovery.

# DAILY SCHEDULE

Use the chart on the next page as a model to develop your daily schedule one week at a time. Block out the times for specific activities and jot down the name of the activity in that block. Include your work, play, and interpersonal activities as well as your recovery activities. You need not account for every minute, but avoid large blocks of unscheduled time. Should such open blocks appear, plan pro-recovery activities for them. Review your plan daily and make adjustments as necessary.

# Daily Schedule

Week of _____

| | Sun. | Mon. | Tues. | Wed. | Thurs. | Fri. | Sat. |
|---|---|---|---|---|---|---|---|
| **AM** 8 | | | | | | | |
| 9 | | | | | | | |
| 10 | | | | | | | |
| 11 | | | | | | | |
| 12 | | | | | | | |
| **PM** 1 | | | | | | | |
| 2 | | | | | | | |
| 3 | | | | | | | |
| 4 | | | | | | | |
| 5 | | | | | | | |
| 6 | | | | | | | |
| 7 | | | | | | | |
| 8 | | | | | | | |
| 9 | | | | | | | |
| 10 | | | | | | | |
| 11 | | | | | | | |

# TWELVE STEP SLOGANS

- Easy does it
- This, too, shall pass
- One day at a time
- First things first
- Turn it over
- Just for today
- Surrender
- More will be revealed
- You're right where you're supposed to be
- Fake it 'til you make it
- You're better than you think you are
- The paralysis of analysis
- Progression not perfection
- Let go and let God
- Stinking thinking
- Only one drink away from a drunk
- Powerless over people, places, and things
- Keep it simple
- God works through people
- Live in the solution not the problem

- Live life on life's terms
- Live in today
- Thy will, not mine
- If you don't take that first drink, you can't get drunk
- One drink is too many, but a thousand are not enough
- Live and let live
- Meeting makers make it